IT'S NOT THAT COMPLICATED

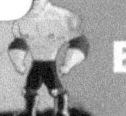

BODYBUILDING FOR DUMBBELLS !

THIS BOOK IS A MUST FOR EVERY BODYBUILDER

By Ric Drasin

CREATOR OF THE 'GOLD'S GYM' AND 'WORLD GYM' LOGO AND FORMER TRAINING PARTNER OF ARNOLD SCHWARZENEGGER and RECIPIENT OF THE 'JOE GOLD LIFETIME ACHIEVEMENT AWARD'

THE GOLDEN ERA TRAINING AND DIET THAT REALLY WORKED TO GIVE US THE GREAT BODIES WE HAD BACK THEN AT VENICE BEACH

Ric Drasin

SIMPLE STEPS TO GREATNESS
TRAINING ROUTINES THAT WORKED
TRAINING PARTNERS THAT HELPED
POSITIVE ATTITUDES IN TRAINING
MUSCLE ENHANCEMENT DRUGS BACK

RICSCORNER.COM

THE RIC SAY'S

RIC DRASIN

Ric is a pioneer of the bodybuilding world since 1960, he then went into professional wrestling in 1965 making a successful career in both sports. Ric was the training partner of Arnold Schwarzenegger during the Golden Era of bodybuilding at Gold's Gym Venice in 1969 and the following years. He designed the famous Gold's Gym t-shirt logo along with the World Gym Gorilla. Ric has been in many issues of Muscle and Fitness magazines along with other publications and started his own bodybuilding t-shirt line in the mid-1970's, the first one in the industry to do so. He has trained many celebrities and professional wrestlers in his ring over the years and has a vast knowledge of both sports.

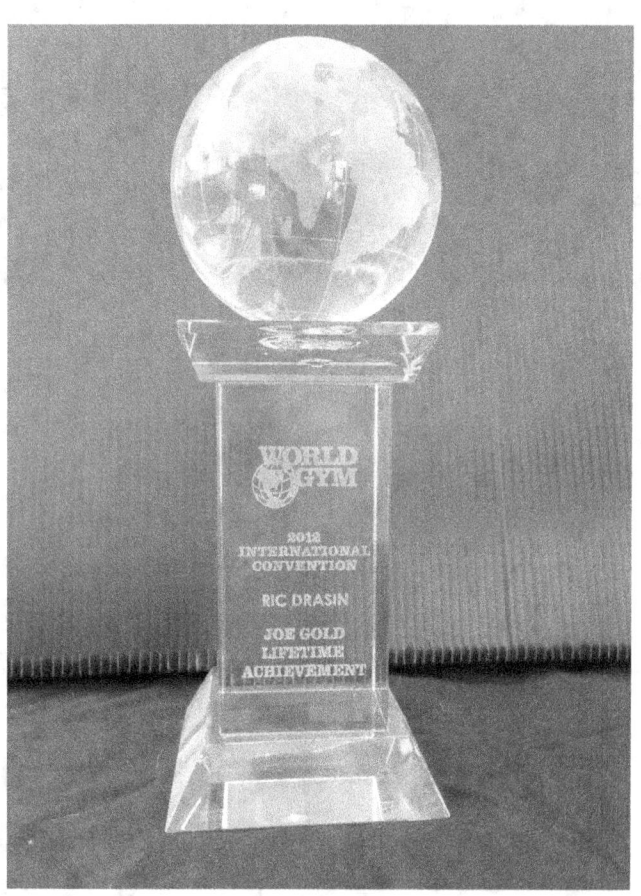

Just recently Ric received the Joe Gold Lifetime Achievement Award in Las Vegas. Now he's sharing his knowledge with you. You can also find him on his own show Ric's Corner which is well over 7 million viewers.

MY START INTO BODYBUILDING

When I was growing up in Bakersfield I got my hands on some body-building magazines as we all did and was inspired about improving myself. I wasn't sure where to begin, as it seemed complicated. How many sets? What do I eat? What do I need for equipment? Since there weren't many gyms around, I started with the basics which back then was a barbeque bench, straight bar and a set of dumbbells which you had to take the collars of and keep changing plates. As you know this can be a pain in the ass but that's all we had back then.

The bench was wood and too wide so it'd rub blisters on my back but I was able to at least do some bench presses but needed a spotter, as there wasn't anywhere to rack the weight.

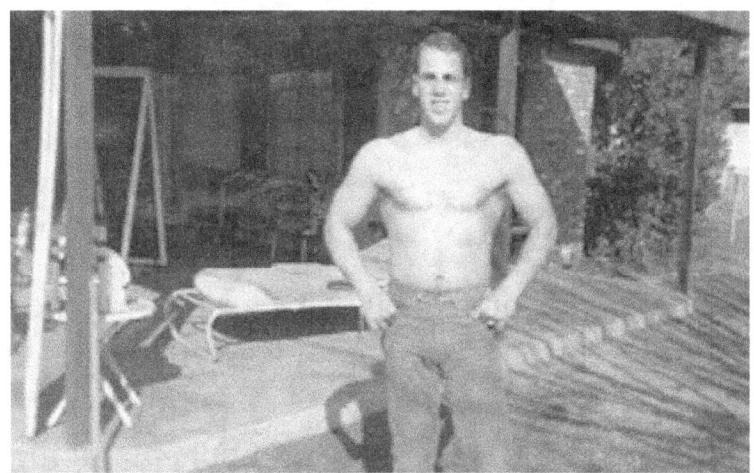

Ric 'The Beginning' 1960

I worked out on my patio and did the basics; bench press, standing press, standing curls, lying triceps, squats and sit ups. That was about it. I read these routines in the magazines with the likes of Steve Reeves who had one of the best bodies around. It said, "workout 3 sets per exercise, 3 times a week." Well, we know today things have changed greatly but I was able to make some gains with that.

My diet consisted of no diet. No one really knew what to eat back then other than vanilla protein pills that tasted like nothing I've ever eaten so I got most my protein from milk, cheese and meat. I wasn't carb conscious but managed to keep my fat low and gained muscle, but then again I was only 17.

I got bored of working out at home and stumbled upon the YMCA that had a weight room. Not a good one but better than the home equipment I was using. At least they had benches, dumbbells to some degree, squat rack and bench press rack.

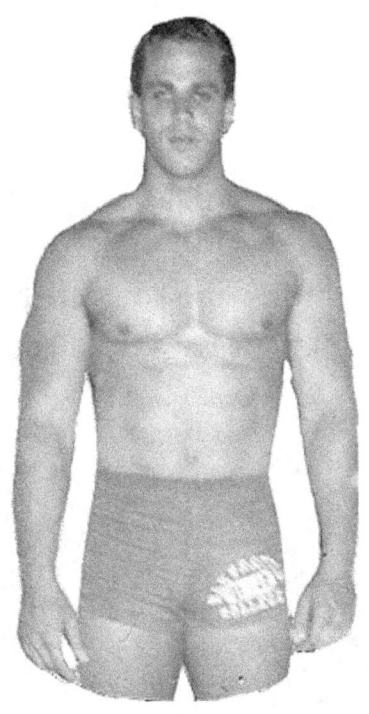

This improved my body quite a bit just after the first month and I was already up to 225 lbs. on the bench and gradually broke 300 lbs. not too far down the road.

I learned to separate body parts by reading the magazines, which made my workouts a whole lot easier. Doing the whole body in one day 3 times a week was hard and took many hours in the gym.

I switched to upper body one day and legs the next and this seemed to be much better but still 3 times a week on everything. The reason this works is because there aren't as many sets and reps on the muscle so they have time to recover in between days.

I was the only one of my friends who wanted to work out and become a bodybuilder. Most thought it was stupid and I took a lot of criticism for doing it but I was focused and that was the key. You have to keep a straight vision of where you see yourself and imagine what you want to look like and shoot for it. Let your mirror talk to you, not the scale. Even though I was gaining weight like mad, my mirror told me where to develop and where to cut back.

These workouts went on for sometime and then I found a better gym in town that really had some updated equipment. The owner was competitive bodybuilder, only 5'5" but had the muscle and proportion so I listened and learned from him. He only trained like 30 to 45 minutes whereas I was putting in 1 ½ hours daily. I was overtraining but you couldn't tell me that. I've seen so many people overtrain and it's really senseless as it destroys the muscle and tears it down way too much. Training isn't building muscle, it's tearing it down and rest and sleep is building it.

I tried to cut back but my mental state kept telling me to do more and more and more. I would sleep more to make up for it though.

From this gym, I moved to another gym down town which wasn't so much chrome and more hardcore. They had the only Olympic bar, which increased my bench press to 400 lbs.

I was not only a bodybuilder but also a power lifter to start, with bench press, squat and deadlift. This gave me the foundation to pack on thick muscle that stayed with me. The heavy lifting gave me the foundation I needed. I just needed to round it off with shaping movements.

While living in Bakersfield at my young age, I used to take a friend or two and drive to Santa Monica beach on some of the weekends to lie out in the sun and hang out at Muscle Beach. This was the original muscle beach before it moved to Venice. My first spotting of Larry Scott really inspired me to train even harder.

I went to a few health food stores in the area, which seemed to have more knowledge of supplements than the ones in my hometown. I learned about some of the vitamins needed and better proteins for better results.

I spoke a lot to some of the less known bodybuilders on the beach to learn and they for sure knew more than I did as they lived in the Mecca of it. We discussed sets and reps, diet, rest, heavy lifting vs. lightweights and I began to change my workout instantly. I also saw changes right away and diet was key in this instance.

Long story short, a few years later I moved to the Los Angeles and began training at Bill Pearls Gym in 1969. Bill was one of the number one bodybuilders and would train at 5 am every morning. Here's where I really learned how to split body parts and not go crazy with overtraining. He was a believer in maybe 4 or 5 sets per exercise and would split up chest with triceps, back with biceps, shoulders with legs and then rotate it from there.

His diet was mainly high protein with a lot of meat back then even though now he's become a vegetarian. There were a lot of big guys there and of course heavy squats and bench press was in order to get big.

This was very inspirational to be with a higher caliber of bodybuilder, which I wasn't used to. It forced me to train harder and I remember super setting standing triceps extensions with forward rope extensions with a maximum pump.

The guys used a milk and egg protein mixed with water and it gave very good results. Diet was hamburger patties and eggs.

I trained there for about a year and then moved on to Gold's Venice when it was just the beginning of the Golden Era. I quickly befriended Arnold, Dave Draper, Franco, Frank Zane to mention a few and we all became great friends.

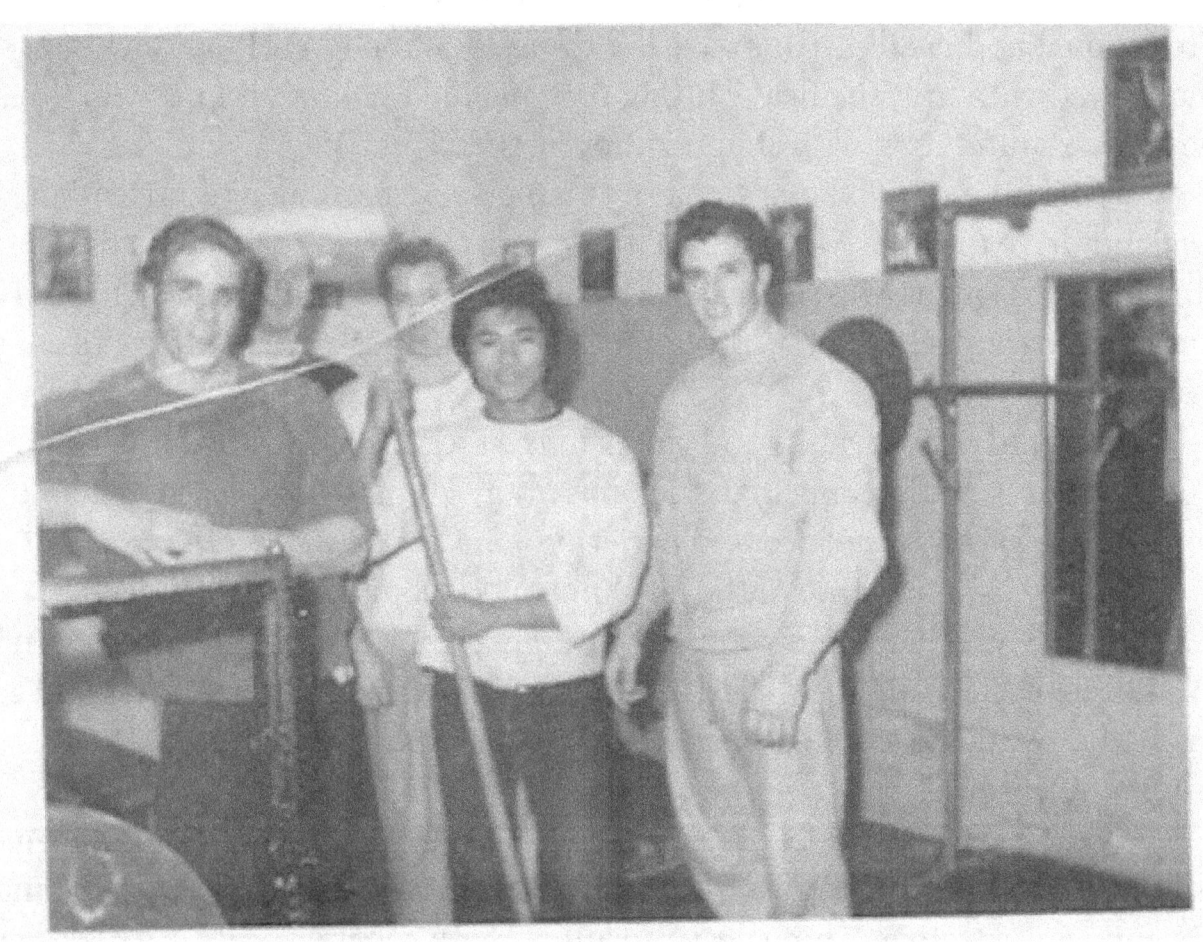

Ric, Gary Johnston, Dave Shambeau

THE WORKOUTS

My training went through changes again and I began to train with Arnold who was a great training partner and we would do chest and back on Monday, which consisted of:

Bench Press 4 sets pyramid up from 225 lbs to 400 lbs. 10, 8, 6, 4, 2 reps
Incline Press usually on the bar 4 sets of pyramids again.
Dumbbell flies 4 sets of 8 reps
Cable crossover 4 sets of 12 reps

Then on to back.

Chins 4 sets of 12 reps
Seated Lat Pulls 4 sets of 8 to 12 reps
One Arm Cable Pulls 4 sets of 8 to 12 reps
Sometimes switch off to T Bars 4 sets of 12 reps
Nautilus Pullover machine 4 sets of 12 reps.

Now this is a basic routine but we all made great progress with this.

Remember, having a good dependable training partner is key for your workouts as you can increase poundage and push each other and it's fun as well.

When at all possible we would change up the workout to supersets such as:

Bench press superset with Chins
Incline superset with T Bar rows
Dumbbell flies superset with Seated Lat Pulls.

This was a great combo for a really good pump. Nothing elaborate but simple and effective.

After that came abs which were leg raises or crunches.

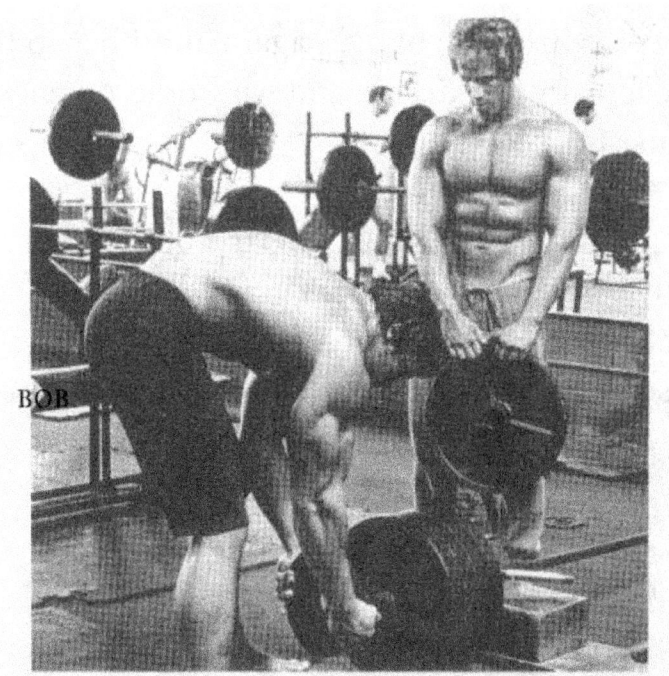

BOB

ARNOLD AND RIC preparing the T-Bar

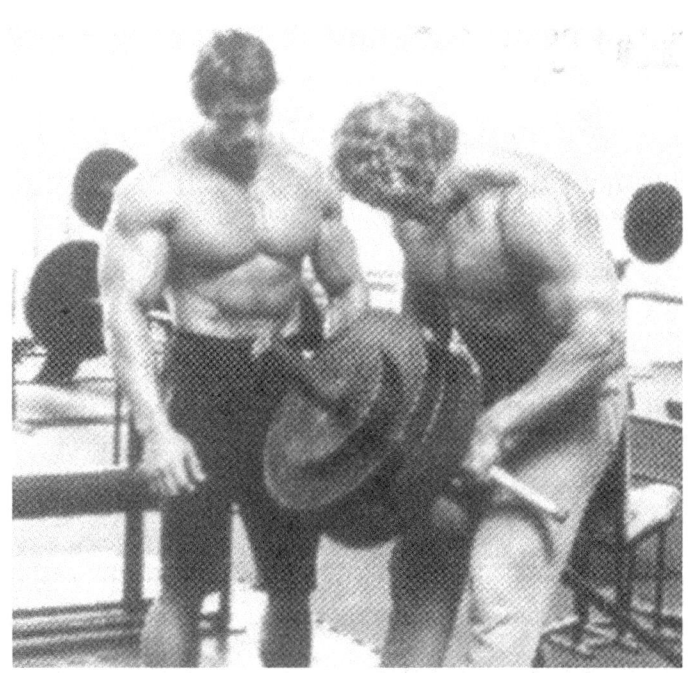

ARNOLD AND RIC doing T-Bar Rows

Next day we did Shoulders and Arms.

Starting with Delts:

We would take the 20 lbs. dumbbells and do the standing twisting dumb-bell presses for 8 reps, then 25 lbs., then 30 lbs. and so on up to 65 lbs. dumb-bells. Then we'd work back down to 20 lbs.

This is a grueling routine but really pumps the delts. After this it was the same up and down the rack with dumbbell lateral raises. That's all we needed for out delt workout and they got real round and thick.

Now as an alternative we would do seated DB presses superset with standing DB laterals. 5 sets 8 reps, graduating up in weight. This is another good system.

You've probably never heard of Tri-sets but that would be adding bent over laterals as the 3rd exercise, so we would rotate between all three move-ments.

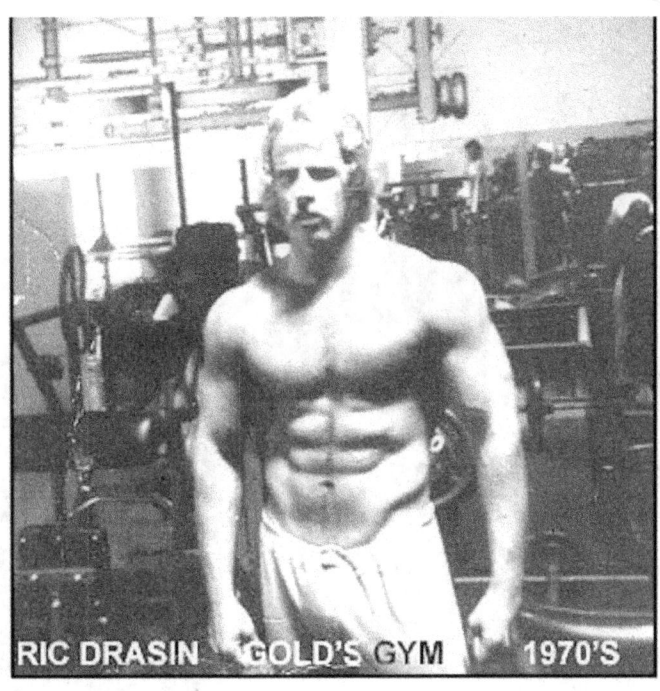

RIC DRASIN   GOLD'S GYM   1970'S

After this we went to Arms.

Usually arms went like this:

Dumbbell curls seated on incline 4 sets 8 reps
Barbell curls 4 sets 8 reps
One arm bent over concentration curls 4 sets 8 reps

This was all the bicep needed.

Triceps were next.

Triceps Pushdown 4 sets 15 reps
Standing One arm dumbbell triceps extension 4 sets of 8
Lying EZ Curl bar extensions 4 sets of 8

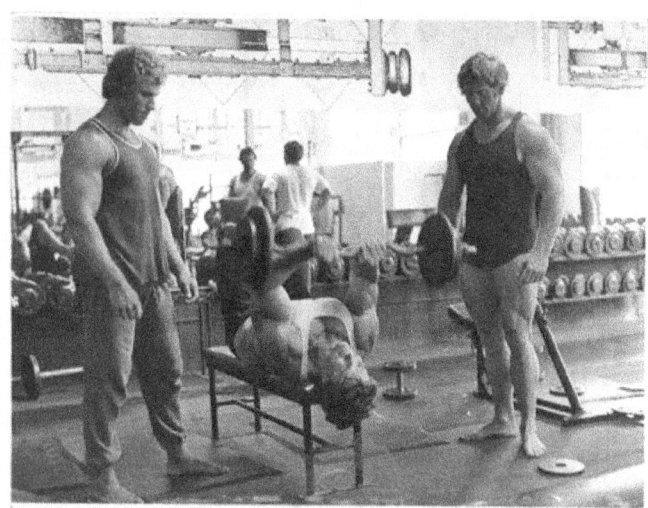

EZ Bar Extensions

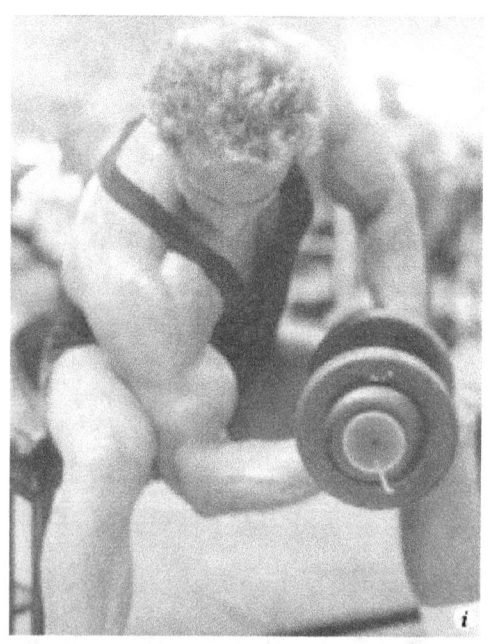

Concentration Curl

Here again, we could sometimes superset. For example,

Standing barbell curl with triceps pushdowns, 4 sets of 8 to 12 reps
Alternate Dumbbell curls with Dumbbell kick backs, 4 sets of 12 reps.
One arm concentration curls seated superset with
One arm behind the neck triceps extensions.

This is another great routine. It's all-basic but simple and works.

Then we get to legs.

I always like to start with calves as it warms up the legs.

Standing calf machine 5 sets of 15 reps for starters,
then I also like Donkey Calf raises (a lost exercise) with two people until failure and then one jumps off and then you finish the reps.

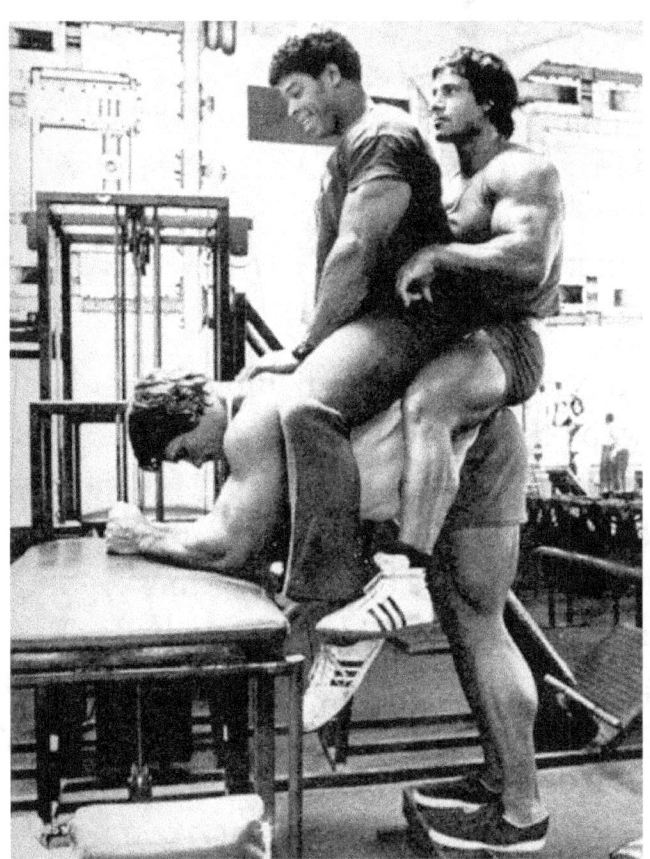

Arnold, Bill Grant and Franco doing donkey calf raises.

After calves, we will go to

Squat – 5 sets of 12, 10, 8, 6, 4 reps.
Leg press 4 sets of 12 reps.
Leg extension 4 set of 12 reps.
Leg curl 5 sets of 12 reps.

This is a really good leg workout that will add size and shape.

Hit 100 abs every day and if you add cardio, only 3 days a week. 20 minutes is plenty, too much cardio eats the muscle.

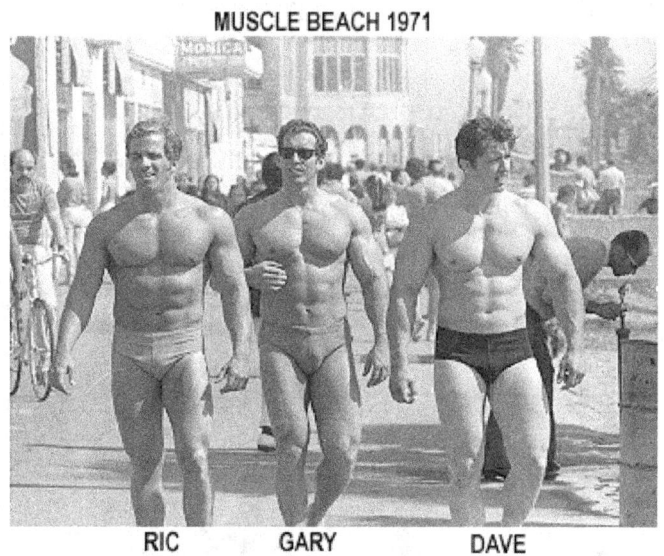

MUSCLE BEACH 1971

RIC   GARY   DAVE

I always felt when I was having a sticking point or getting nowhere in my workout, it was back to basics. I've done as many as 25 sets for biceps and as little as 8. Recently I found that I got more out of the 8 sets than I did 25 sets. I was over training them and they weren't responding.

We would train 6 days a week and sometimes 7 going in on Sunday and hitting some odd exercises that we didn't normally do. This brought good results as well. For a period of time I trained with Bill Grant and we did a 4-day routine with 3 days off. This was also very good for growth as those off days did a lot of good to repair the muscle.

These routines were not complicated back then. We knew what body part we wanted to work and we worked it. We knew how to flush and pump the muscle to max size and growth.

I see so many people in the gyms today who have no clue how to train. I used to offer to help and some are receptive and some not. One young trainer asked me once if I wanted him to train me. I just looked at him and thought, if you only knew.

It's also sad today that if you asked most in the gym or even in a Gold's Gym if they know who Joe Gold is. They don't! They have no knowledge that he was the owner, the pioneer of bodybuilding and Gold's Gyms and World Gyms.

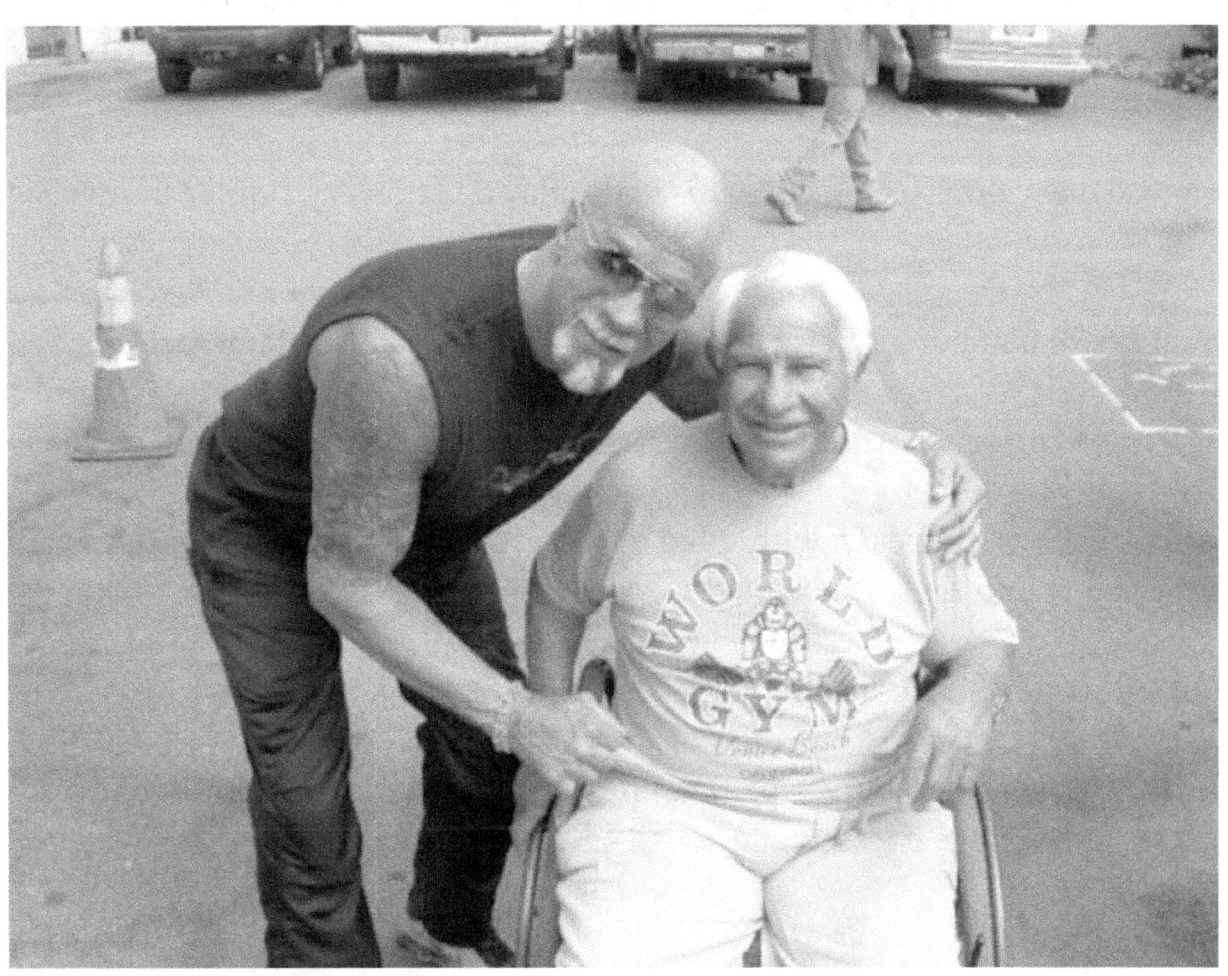

Ric Drasin and Joe Gold

THE DIET

So basically those are the workouts that worked then and still work today. Today's younger bodybuilder in many cases have no respect for those who set the bar and laid the groundwork for bodybuilding. Many eat crazy diets and stuff down any drug they can find. We never did that and now I'm getting to the diet end of it.

The best diet that I found was the diet that we used back in the 70's. It was simple and it worked. Basically high protein and low carbs. Bodybuilders had been using this since the 1940's. Later in years Dr. Atkins put his name on it and then it became the Zone diet, Beverly Hills diet and so on but basically it was a bodybuilding diet without all the fancy names.

In those days it was usually like this and today it's still very similar for me:

Breakfast – hamburger patty with 4 eggs and a scoop of cottage cheese.

Mid-morning snack would be either scrambled eggs or a can of tuna.

Lunch- varied, ½ chicken with salad and veggies with cottage cheese or again burger patty and eggs.

Mid-afternoon snack maybe a chicken breast or two and or tuna.

Dinner- grill a steak, burger patties, chicken, fish your choice with salad and veggies and cottage cheese.

Cottage cheese is a good source of protein and we all made nice gains on this diet.

Now it's up to the individual but some people added more carbs in way of rice or pasta. I preferred to stay lean and did not. I would take fiber at bedtime though as I thought it was important.

Today's diet has changed a bit with oatmeal added in the morning and maybe rice at lunch and dinner. I feel as I get a little older that I need the carb energy. I also added a protein drink with water and fiber at bedtime, which allows it to feed my body as I sleep.

We did have a junk day on Sundays and anything goes all day. You could go crazy on pizza, ice cream, cookies, etc as it went right through your body in one day and you couldn't get fat off of it.

There are more fast food places today that will be health conscious and you can order accordingly to suit your diet so that's a big difference from back in the day. Also we didn't have any really good protein supplements. They were just coming out so it was limited however today there's an abundance of good quality protein and aminos out there.

We took handfuls of liver pills instead. This is a maintenance diet and keeps me at a consistent 225 lbs. It's used to stay in shape and stay lean. If I wanted to get bigger, I would up my carbs and protein and then I would gain size. This is a good all round diet for staying in shape.

You can have one cheat day and eat anything you want. It'll help you keep your sanity.

This is a maintenance diet and keeps me at a consistent 225 lbs. It's used to stay in shape and stay lean. If I wanted to get bigger, I would up my carbs and protein and then I would gain size. This is a good all round diet for staying in shape.

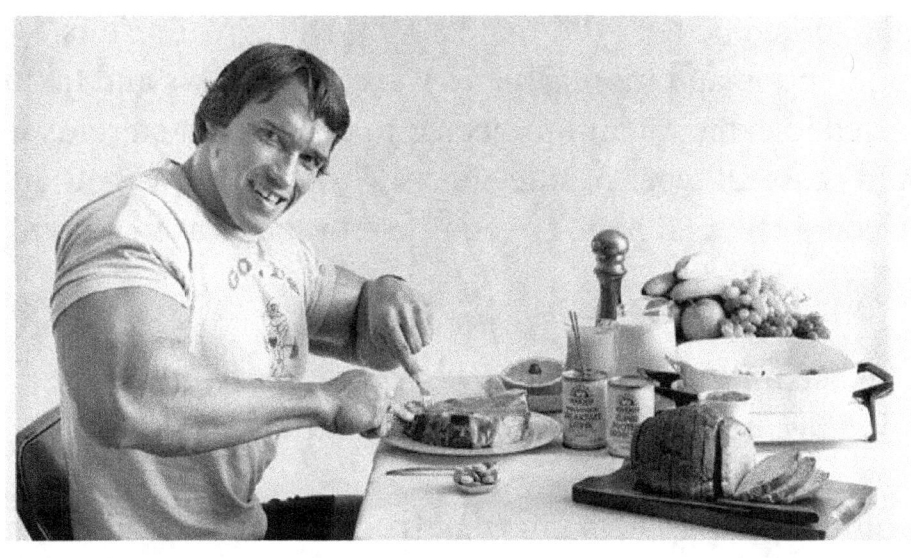

STEROIDS

This was a period long before steroids came about so everything was done naturally. I didn't know any difference and was bench-pressing close to 400 lbs. The good thing about that was it gave me a good foundation that I never lost after that. So many people want the quick way to the top and then you lose it just as fast. I even entered a power lifting contest and took second. I had a bench press then of 425 lbs., squat 510 lbs., deadlift of 575 lbs. and weighed 202 lbs. That was very good for those days.

But steroids did come into play later for me. I had a friend that kept telling me about Dianabol and that Bill Pearl used it for contests. He looked awesome and I had reached plateaus so I felt that maybe I'd try it. I never heard of side effects and figured that it would only enhance my body. I was able to get a bottle from my pharmacist for $8 per 100 tabs. I took 2 a day for a month and I gained about 10 lbs. and got a terrific pump. My arms looked full and I was on my way to a better body. I had no side effects that I could see, not even a pimple.

I cycled on and off and then switched to Winstrol, which actually made me more cut up and harder. It also made my skin like silk. I stuck with tablets and didn't get into the injectables until later. I went from Winstrol to Maxibolan and then Anavar. Each one had it's own effect and made the muscle respond a little different. I think Dianabol was the best for size and strength. It also increased my appetite. I was on meat and cheese diet and it worked but I think that if I would have been more advanced and tightened up on the carbs, it would have worked better. I did that later on with great results.

As time went on and more athletes were in the news and taking steroids, the news started to exploit it and projected to people that steroids were bad for you and could cause all types of side effects. However it was new and there was no way they could tell, as it hadn't been proven yet and at that point it was still legal.

Don't take steroids! Steroids kill. They cause cancer, make your hair fall out, cause 'roid rage, make your chin grow, and more!

Some of these claims are somewhat true but in the hands of the media, steroids have been branded as the devil's evil drug.

Steroids were first used to heal wounded soldiers in World War II for their ability to regenerate damaged tissue. Steroids also fought disease, added recovery strength and gave a mental boost to the injured.

I felt great, in fact, never better. I used them for about 2 months before tapering off. About 1 month later, I dropped 4 pounds, but retained at least 10 pounds. I was ahead of where I was before I started using steroids. I had also increased my metabolism and cut body fat, which made me feel and look much, much harder. I still had fantastic abs.

It wasn't until I moved to Los Angeles and Venice, CA that I was introduced to more advanced, injectable steroids, such as Primo Bolan Depot from Germany. This was injected weekly in conjunction with Dianabol.

Everyone at Gold's Gym in the 70's was taking this combination. Everything was easy to get and really cheap. In the 80's, technology advanced beyond steroids to GH

I tried GH, too. I ignored the recommendation to increase caloric intake to 7,000 a day, so it ripped me up to where I had veins popping on top of veins. In only 10 days, my incline press jumped from 90 to 150 pounds using dumbbells.

Today, chemical technology has become so sophisticated that you need a chemistry degree to know what to take and that's what the Olympia competitors are studying. These guys spend over $75,000 a year just to compete. Honestly, I believe that if you are going to compete at that level, then you need to take them. It will never change. No drug-free competitor will ever be able to measure up against someone who is on the juice and no one will ever achieve such muscularity without drugs unless he is a genetic freak of nature

Steroids can make your hair fall out. An overload of testosterone can block hair growth. Big muscles -- bald head. I don't care. I prefer a bald head. Steroids are now considered a class III drug and are illegal.

The government wants to limit and control our muscle size. Roid rage? Sure, an overdose of hormone can change your mood. So do birth control pills. And PMS -- what's the difference? Be aware of your mood swings. Roid rage can be controlled. It's just an excuse to be an asshole as PMS is to be a bitch.

Doctors now prescribe testosterone for men over 40 to compensate for the body's failure to produce it, which causes hair loss, aging and loss of sex drive. Research in older men shows that test therapy reverses these problems. Testosterone is even being used to fight AIDS and it's working. Growth hormone is also reversing the aging process. In all my years, the worst side effect I have ever seen from steroids is a pimple and a headache. And we would get those anyway. Since you can overdo anything, everything should be done in moderation and monitored by a doctor. The extreme bodybuilder who thinks that if 1 cc a week is good, then 1 cc a day is great, is asking for trouble -- just like taking too many aspirins, or drinking too much or overeating.

I am in no way advocating the use of steroids. If you can do without them, more power to you. If you are not competing or in the public eye, which demands specific sizes and shapes, then stay away from them. My point is that steroids have gotten a bum rap and every idiot on the streets thinks he is an expert because of sensationalist articles in the newspaper. Seems like what ever people read in the paper makes them think that it's got to be true, not realizing that it's just an opinion. And opinions are like assholes. Everyone has one!

I still take test on certain cycles. At 69, my body doesn't produce it anymore. I also take GH which is an anti-aging hormone that really works. I was tested by my Doctor and he wrote me a prescription for Testosterone and Arimadex.

I get pegged for 51 and sometimes even younger. Maybe this is why, or maybe not, but I feel good and have no ailments from them I will say that over use does have a side effect. It can weaken tendon tissue and make it a bit like swiss cheese. Now, I'm not sure how much it takes, but it does happen. It can also be from the muscles getting so strong and the tendons not being able to handle the weight. You hear a lot about torn biceps, pecs, triceps and even quads. This is most likely due to steroids allowing you to go heavier than your tendons can handle.

I have had a lot of injuries from bodybuilding and mostly wrestling. I tore both quads out on my legs and had them reattached. I was a fairly heavy squatter at one time but also wrestling was hell on the knees. My doctor said that some of this is caused by steroids and tendon damage. However testosterone can also be used to repair the same injury as it is now along with GH. So, I'm just giving you the facts. You are the judge and if you should do it, do it in moderation.

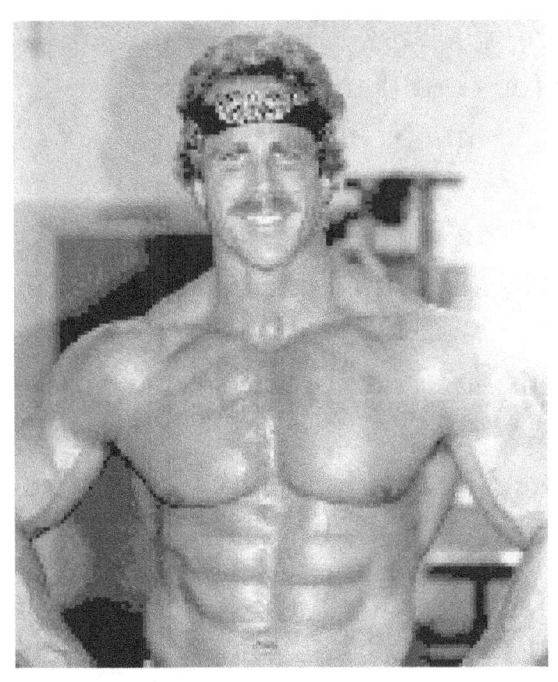

Ric Drasin in the 1980's.

Ric Drasin at 69.

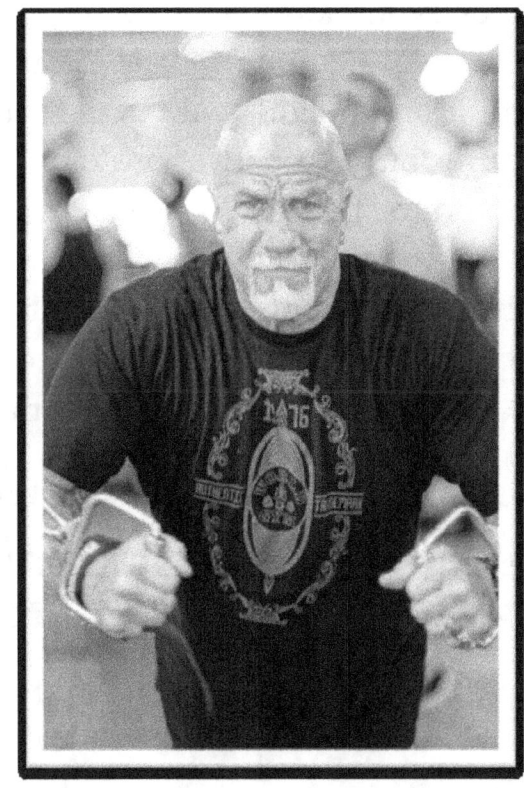

DO'S AND DON'TS OF BODYBUILDING

Do's

- Train with intensity. Make sure every rep counts up and down.
- Every workout should be your best work out. No excuses.
- Limit you time in between sets to around 45 seconds.
- Flush out each body part before going to the next body part.
- Have a system in mind when you go into the gym. Keeping in mind you're routine.
- Alternate exercises and if one machine is busy, don't wait, find another alternative.
- Divide your bodyparts up in groups as far as 2 per day. It works best and this will also give you each part twice a week.
- 3 to 4 exercises per bodypart. Reps can vary and sets 3 to 4. I've found lately that less is more and do 3 sets per exercise whereas I used to do 5 sets per exercise.
- Finish up with abs and cardio. Best done at the end of the workout so that you can focus on the sets.
- Take one meal at a time and eat clean. Don't worry about tomorrow's meals, they'll come around and you can plan then.
- Make sure you get plenty of protein throughout the day. This means about every few hours. It feeds your muscle.
- You can have carbohydrates when training hard but remember everyone's metabolism is different. If you hold fat on your body and in the muscle then cut the carbs. This is old school but it works.
- Keep a positive attitude towards training and life in general. Everything reflects on your well being. Bad attitude, means bad day means bad workout.
- Treat everyone in the gym with respect and you'll get it back twice over.
- <u>Don't drop your weights and put them back when done.</u> This is courtesy in the gym.

Don't's

- Don't eat refined sugars if you want to develop a good body. I stay away from white, meaning potatoes, rice, white flour, white sugar, pasta. Now there are exceptions of coure as events and parties come up and you have to partake in some of this, but not on a steady basis. Sushi is OK once in awhile with the rice.
- Don't throw the weights up and down. Focus on the muscle. Mirrors are good and the reason for them is to watch the body in motion and doing the work correct.
- Don't come to the gym in smelly workout wear. This is a heavy breathing sport and it's offensive to smell some one bad or bad breath when training. I've seen this a number of times and people get kicked out for it. Poor hygiene.
- Don't over indulge in alcohol if you want to put on good muscle as it tears cells down and slows recovery.
- Don't over do your cardio when trying to build muscle. Lots of cardio burns muscle too.
- Don't get lazy and miss workouts. It's so easy not to hit the gym and I've found out, once I'm there and do a couple of sets, I feel better. My whole mood changes.
- Don't overdose on steroids or any other drug for that matter. If you choose to use them, then do it in moderation under a doctor's care. Don't be foolish and ruin your life over having an 18" arm.

Ric say's:

Don't ever give up or lose confidence in yourself. There's only one of you in this world and you're unique and valuable to us. So be the best you that you can be. We love you and need you in our world!

This pretty much simplifies bodybuilding and I hope it helps you reach your goals. Stay tuned to Ric's Corner for more info and eat healthy, train hard, and grow to your hearts content. I'm always here for you, so carry on the torch for us!

-Ric Drasin 2013

Websites

RICDRASIN.COM
RICSCORNER.COM - Host
ACTORSENTERTAINMENT.COM   - Host
AFTERBUZZTV.COM – Host

Sponsors

http://www.anabolicoutlaws.com

http://www.worldgym.com

http://www.goldsgym.com

http://www.paceboss.com

http://www.nutrifit.com

http://www.prowrestlingdreams.com

http://www.actorsentertainment.com

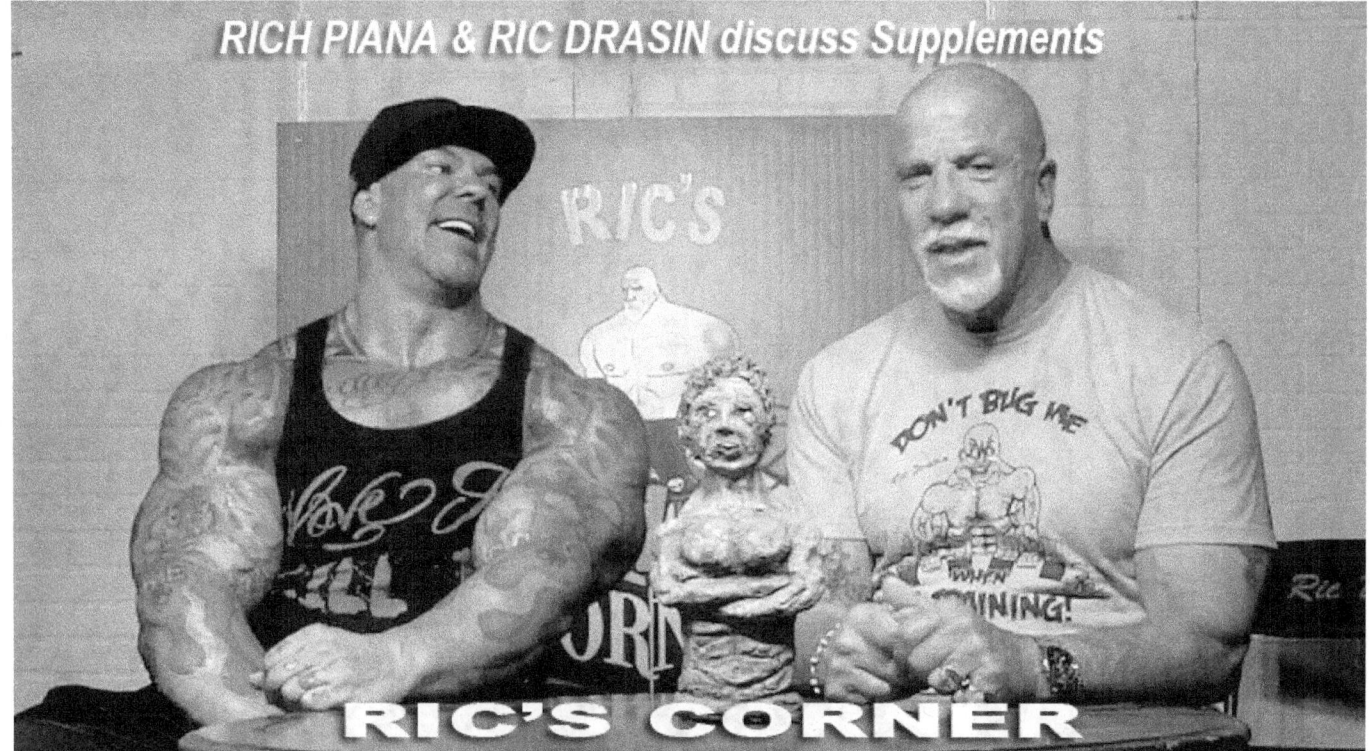

RICH PIANA & RIC DRASIN discuss Supplements

RIC'S

RIC'S CORNER

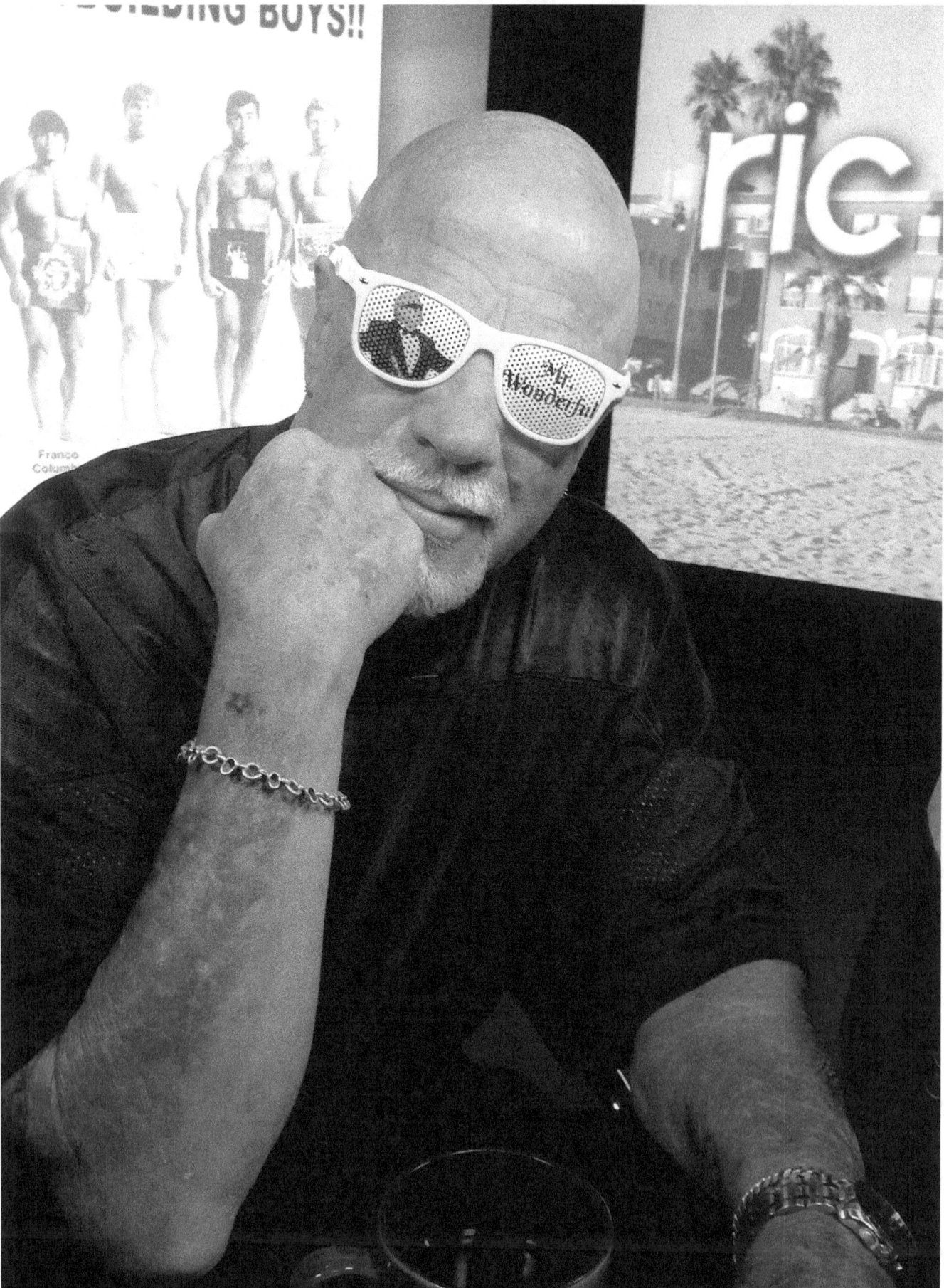

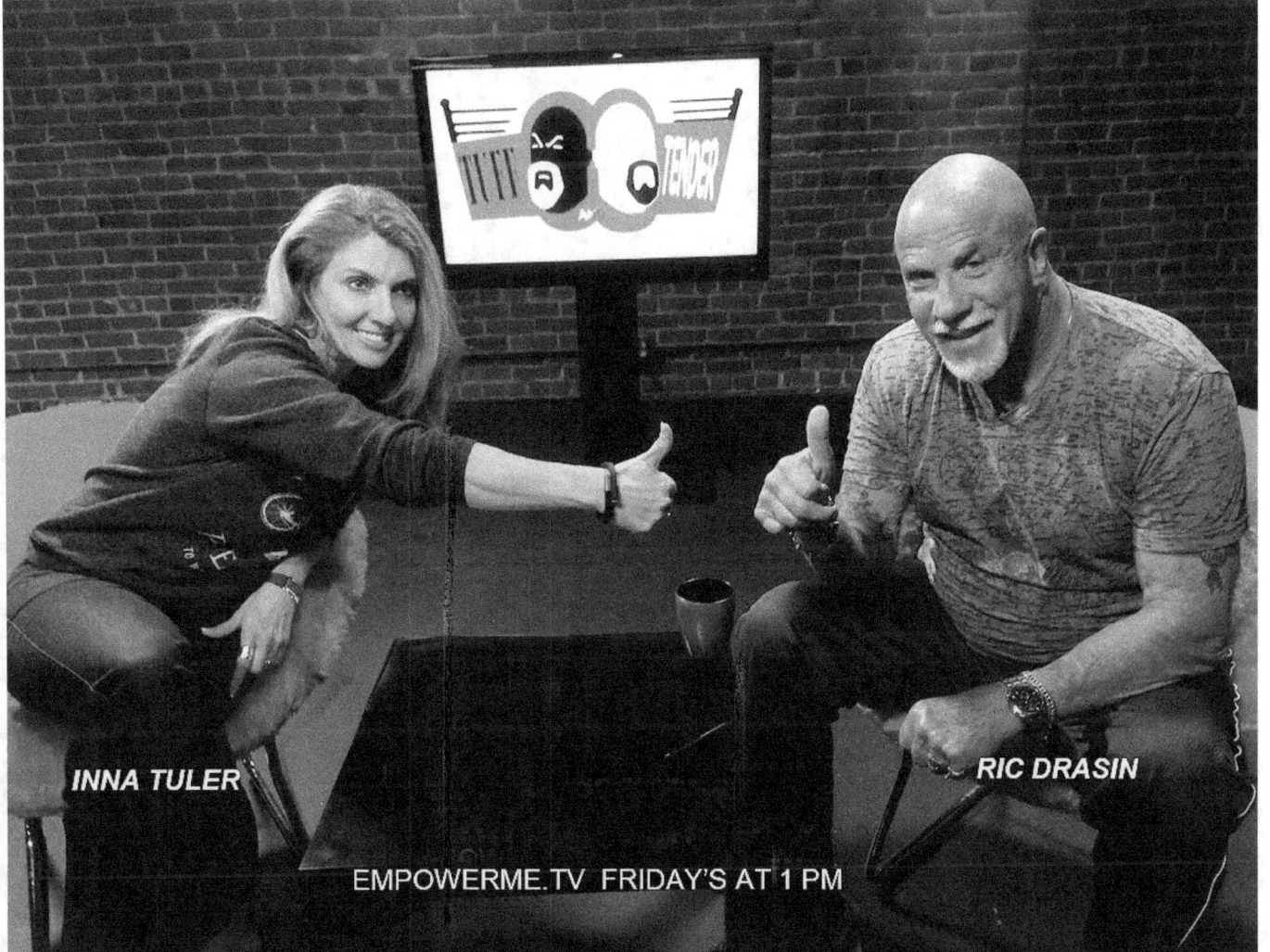

INNA TULER

RIC DRASIN

EMPOWERME.TV FRIDAY'S AT 1 PM

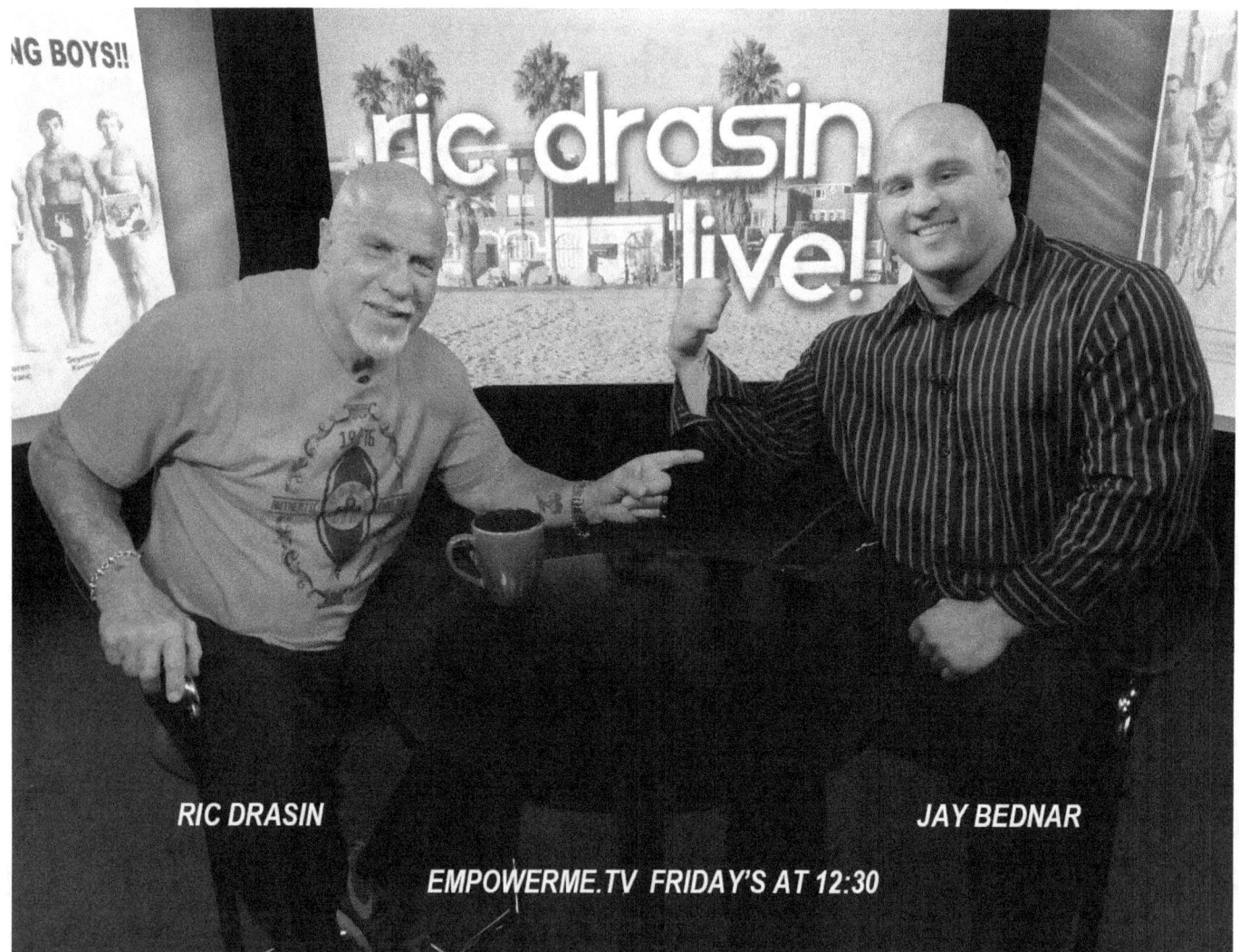

RIC DRASIN   JAY BEDNAR

EMPOWERME.TV FRIDAY'S AT 12:30